P[RE]-INVENT

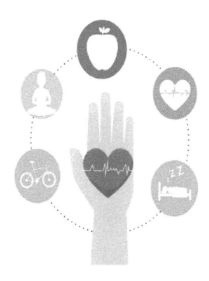

By

STEVE SHUCH RN, BSN, CNOR

TABLE OF CONTENTS

PREFACE

This book has taken me over ten years from concept to publication. Each time I researched and started writing, I realized that healthcare had evolved. We have transitioned from treating illness to preventing it! Dynamic, functional, and inclusive healthcare is what we are working towards and will be the way of the future. Reinventing how we look at our health and healthcare will lead to sickness prevention and help promote longevity. Incorporating Artificial Intelligence (AI) within the multidisciplinary team, the consumer (patient), eating habits, and proper nutrition supplementation are all equally crucial for total health and well-being.

Throughout the years, I have gained knowledge and collected information through many experiences that have led me to the here and now. This guide will discuss multiple ideas backed by many years of research. One thing to remember is that healthcare is linked to technology! Both are ever-changing, with results to improve the functionality of life as we know it!

Part 1 of this guide will make you ponder what your health and well-being mean to you. I hope you enjoy and learn from this guide, as I have enjoyed writing it!

Also, please remember to "Live, Love, Learn, and Teach!"

CHAPTER 1

Health and Wellness

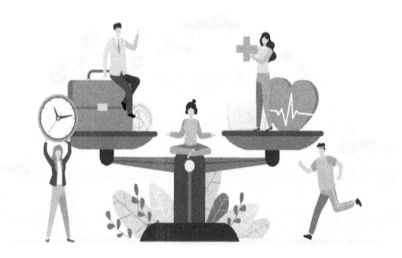

We hear the terms "Health and Wellness" almost everywhere we go. At just about any age, people are talking about it. Health and wellness is everywhere. Parents talk to their toddlers about Health and Wellness; even places like MyGym educate parents regarding recommended foods for their toddlers. Then, at the opposite end of the spectrum, we have an aging population looking for longevity through anti-aging medicines, looking into telomeres, and taking Silver Sneakers classes.

The World Health Organization (WHO) defines health as complete physical, mental, and social well-being, not merely the absence of disease or infirmity. Our health is essential because if our health starts to deteriorate, a façade of effects may happen. For instance, when faced with health concerns, we ask ourselves, "How am I going to cope with taking care of family stressors?" Also, when we are on an airplane, we are told in an emergency to place the oxygen on ourselves first, before helping others. Thus, our health must be our 1st priority because we are of no help if we are unhealthy.

Health also comes in many formats: physical, mental, spiritual, emotional, and financial. All these factors can affect our overall health. Psychological and physical health, are two of the most important factors for overall health.

Mental health not only pertains to those with mental disorders but all of us. Mental health refers to a person's emotional, social, and psychological well-being; mental health is as important as physical health to an active lifestyle (Felman, 2017). Daily stressors will affect one's mental health, and one's ability to learn stress-reducing methods (techniques), whether from meditation, guided imagery, or whatever means, will help strengthen mental health.

Physical health is not necessarily about how much weight you lift or how strong you are. It is about overall fitness! The European Patients Academy states, "Physical health is defined as the condition of your body, considering everything from the absence of disease to fitness level." One's physical health is vital for overall well-being. Our physical health can be affected by many aspects of our life. Genetics may play a part and can make achieving physical health challenging.

A recent study published in the journal *PLOS ONE* and led by experts from the Cambridge Centre for Sport & Exercise Sciences at Anglia Ruskin University (ARU) in England found that up to 72% of the difference between people in performance outcome following a specific exercise can be due to genetic differences. These differences include muscle strength, cardiovascular fitness, and anaerobic power.

Our environment also plays a role. For instance, people who work in the sun have increased risk for skin cancer and toxic substance inhalation. With over a million cases of skin cancers diagnosed annually, many could be prevented by protecting the skin from excessive sun exposure and not using indoor tanning devices.

Most importantly, it comes down to lifestyle choices! One's nutrition (diet), level of exercise, and social decisions, like tobacco use and alcohol consumption, will majorly alter one's physical health. Nutritional choice, such as increasing fiber-rich foods, may reduce the chance of colon cancer by over twenty percent. In contrast, a lifestyle choice, such as regular alcohol consumption, can increase the chances of colon cancer. Also, a lifestyle choice like cigarette smoking is linked to lung cancer. The *association between tobacco cigarette smoking and lung cancer is well established*, but smoking is also highly harmful to the colon and rectum. Evidence shows that 12% of colorectal cancer deaths are attributed to smoking (Sawicki et al., 2021).

Additionally, one disease that is considered a lifestyle disease is Type II diabetes. Age, obesity, and diet are the main culprits causing Type II diabetes; besides age, both are modifiable risk factors. Persons diagnosed with diabetes or pre-diabetes can change these modifiable risk factors to manage their diabetes and lower blood glucose levels. These modifiable risk factors include altering their diet by choosing healthier choices, increasing exercise, and eliminating unhealthy lifestyle activities (e.g., smoking, excessive alcohol, insufficient sleep) (Boles, Kandimalla, & Reddy, 2017).

Wellness and health differ as much as they are similar. University of California, Davis, defines wellness as "An active process of becoming aware of and making choices toward a healthy and fulfilling life; it is more than being free from illness. It is a dynamic process of change and growth." Wellness is the act of being healthy. This is where we go from treating illness to preventing, from feeling better to flourishing, basically "Reinventing Healthcare!"

As with health, we can break down wellness into subcategories. This is where health and fitness have similar ideas, just different actions. Physical wellness focuses on obtaining a healthy body through exercise, adequate rest, and proper nutrition. Mental (emotional and intellectual) focuses on having an open mind to potentially new ideas, continuing to learn, understanding one's feelings, and relating and coping with stress. As I mentioned in the Preface, remember to "**Live, Love, Learn, and Teach!**"

UC Davis States: "Maintaining an optimal level of wellness is crucial to living a higher quality life. Wellness matters. Wellness matters because everything we do and every emotion we feel relates to our well-being. In turn, our well-being directly affects our actions and emotions. It's an ongoing circle. Therefore, everyone needs to achieve optimal wellness to subdue stress, reduce the risk of illness, and ensure positive interactions."

CHAPTER 2

HEALTHCARE AS WE KNOW IT

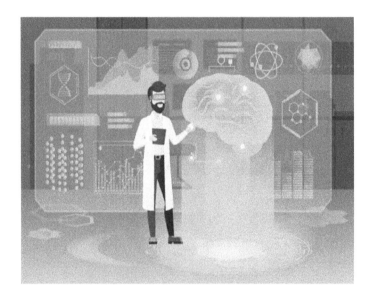

Healthcare is currently undergoing a paradigm, shift from treating to preventing illness. Historically, one would go to the doctor when suffering from an ailment. Whether you had a cold, flu, or something even more severe, these were the only times to go to the Doctor. Now, we have more options to see a doctor, and physician extenders are more prevalent and trusted. Physician assistants and nurse practitioners are picking up where physicians leave off. We can reach more patients and at an increased pace. Healthcare now offers urgent care locations and even telemedicine (telehealth), such as online applications where you can see the healthcare provider face-to-face. These options are helping to create a more accessible healthcare system. However, we are still missing the point! Accessibility is important, but the focus needs to be on a dynamic and functional approach to health and wellness.

Today, healthcare has shifted to more prevention, offering community health options and highly recommended yearly physicals, including health and wellness check-ups. Most insurance companies even give discounts when we are proactive with our healthcare. Many companies provide discounts for annual physicals, being tobacco-free, and even for receiving the flu vaccine. Insurance companies, however, dictate too much of the costs, reducing the time doctors must see patients while increasing the patient load. This can prevent the doctor from building a positive relationship with their patients because the patient is reduced to becoming "a number." This needs to change!

Our healthcare is not inadequate, yet it could be much better. It is not all doom and gloom; our healthcare system is still one of the best. We have fantastic healthcare providers using cutting-edge technologies to treat and cure patients. Overall, people are healthier, doing better financially, and living longer today than 30 years ago (Durrani, 2016). What can we do to live a healthier, improved quality life? Think about this quote by Dr. Seuss, "It is not about what it is, but about what it can become!"

CHAPTER 3

ESTABLISHING YOUR DEFINITION OF HEALTH AND WELLNESS

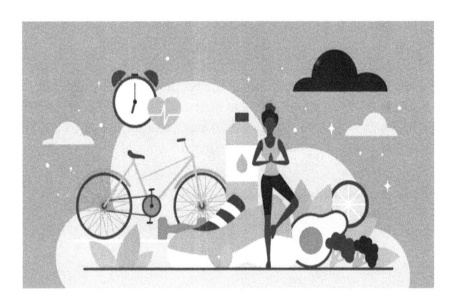

W hy? I know what health and wellness is to me! In a nutshell, it is to see my daughter prosper into a wonderful adult. I want to be healthy enough to play catch with potential grandchildren and care for my family well into my late years. I cannot say if there is a fountain of youth, but I will do my best to help offset the aging process. Whether through lifestyle changes, meditation, proper supplementation, and/or hormone replacement, I am prepared to go all-in on my longevity. Health and wellness goals may differ from person to person; what we are trying to achieve is what "quality of life" will be for you.

• What does this mean to you?

• How do you feel about your overall health?

• What about wellness? Are you actively trying to reduce stressors and create an optimal lifestyle?

• When did you last have a health check-up or mental health break?

• What are you currently doing to create peace in your life?

• As it pertains to your health, where do you see yourself in 5 years, 10 years, or even 20?

• What are you doing to help you get there/change your paradigm?

• What are your overall health and wellness goals?

These are all great questions; think about them for a moment. Write them down, answer them, and tweak them as necessary. This information will be vital in helping you to reinvent your health and wellness.

CHAPTER 4

REINVENT TO PREVENT!

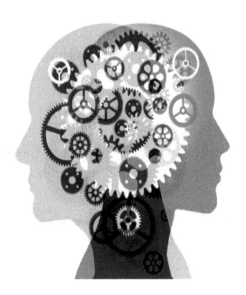

As I mentioned previously, a dynamic, functional, and inclusive healthcare system is what we are working toward. This means we need to reinvent healthcare! We need to create a systematic approach within the health and wellness communities. The concept of systemness is a newer approach in healthcare. Systemness means interconnected or integrating all aspects of health and wellness.

One centralized and cohesive plan to prevent illness and promote wellness can help increase the overall quality of life. This new multidisciplinary team will be based on respecting and understanding each other's specialty. This approach could be considered holistic, but it includes all aspects of health and wellness, with the overall goal of living our best life!

Dynamic or constantly changing healthcare is a must. Keeping up with research and technology and not fearing change is essential to health and wellness. If a medical provider is not willing to look at the newest information and technology, do they have your best interest at hand?

Functional medicine is an approach that focuses on establishing the root cause of the illness. Furthermore, functional medicine represents an operational system that focuses on the underlying causes of disease from a systems biology perspective that engages the patient and practitioner in a therapeutic partnership (Jones, 2010). Each ailment is caused by something. For example, an inflammatory response can cause heart disease, arthritis, diabetes, etc. What caused the inflammation? Was it a vitamin deficiency or lack of rest? See the connection between health and wellness? But wait, there's more….

Applying a dynamic approach to functional medicine, such as new research into the benefits of Omega-3 fatty acids and the reduction of inflammation, shows the use of systemness. Omega-3 fatty acids can reduce the production of molecules and substances linked to inflammation, such as inflammatory eicosanoids and cytokines. The reduction of cytokines directly helps those who have asthma.

Are doctors the best resource for nutritional supplements? NO! However, they are essential in understanding how one supplement may be contraindicated with another or how it will affect a medication you may be on. Systemness is crucial, with a proper understanding of medications, supplements, and how they are intertwined.

Creating this inclusiveness, incorporating many different specialists by combining the needs of the individual, is a must in promoting prevention! The patient must have a voice; understanding their goals is only part of the equation. The need to be healthy is there, but how will we get to where we want to be?

In Chapter 3, you wrote down some goals and ideas about your quality of life. Discuss these with your healthcare provider (ask your provider for inputs on action plans that can assist you in succeeding; just an idea here). Discuss an action plan to help you succeed. Many functional medicine doctors have or work with other clinicians, such as health coaches and nutritional professionals. Also, if needed, many online wellness programs can be used to help one stay focused on the prize!

CHAPTER 5

EATING HEALTHY AND PROPER SUPPLEMENTATION

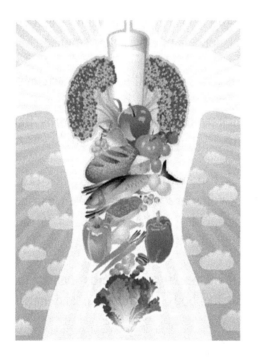

Health and wellness come in many categories, such as physical, mental, and even spiritual, that affect us.

In this chapter, we will discuss the basics of eating healthy and utilizing proper supplementation, as this is the longest and most important part of prevention. As mentioned earlier, finding the root cause of ailments is a must. Most root causes are those relating to inadequate nutrition and supplementation. This is a challenging chapter to write, for there is so much information that I would like to share.

As you notice, I don't use the term "diet" because we think of fads when we think of diets! Eating healthy is a lifestyle change. There is no "one size fits all" plan for eating healthy. This is your body; you must pay attention to what your body is telling you! Everyone is different and metabolizes food in their own way. Luckily, if we want to take it a step further, food allergen tests are available to see what foods you may be sensitive to.

If you're looking to lose weight, it is based on calories in, versus out. This is basic math. Have I told you that I love math? Math is accurate, and it is absolute! I also love science, and nutrition is science.

Nutrition is defined as the "science of food, the nutrients and other substances therein, their action, interaction, and balance about health and disease, and the processes by which the organism ingests, absorbs, transports, utilizes and excretes food substances" (Lagua & Claudio, 2012).

Nutrition can be broken down into macronutrients: proteins, carbohydrates (Carbs), and fats. Proteins are amino acids that can be broken down into branched-chain amino acids (BCAAs) and essential amino acids (EAAs), which are protein's building blocks.

Our body creates 10 of the 20 amino acids that are needed. BCAAs and EAAs are those that the body cannot make and must come from a food source.

Carbs include fiber, sugars, starches, and a 4th group of oligosaccharides (fall between starch and sugar). The last group is that of fats. We mostly think fat is wrong, but that is not always true! Fats are broken down into good unsaturated (monounsaturated fats and polyunsaturated fats), bad saturated fats, and the worst, trans fatty acids (trans fat). Nutrition also incorporates micronutrients of minerals and vitamins.

So, what is good nutrition? With so many different ideas ("diets") from intermittent fasting, Keto, Mediterranean, South Beach, and many more, you may be wondering, what is the "best "way to eat? As I mentioned, you know your body; listen to it! Kaiser Permanente recommends more fruits, low-fat dairy, vegetables, and whole grains. In addition, consider purchasing a healthy recipe book. Not too helpful?

Cleveland Clinic's website has tips on how to spot a fad diet. It is a fad if it promises a quick fix based on a single study and states to eliminate one or more food groups.

Cleveland Clinic suggests, "The best method to lose weight and keep it off is to exercise regularly and eat a variety of foods with moderate portions." As I mentioned before, this is not a one-size-fits-all type of deal!

To eat healthily, we must understand what we put in our bodies. Our bodies work efficiently when fed moderate portions more often throughout the day. I recommend 5-6 smaller meals spread throughout the day. Protein is essential for our bodies to function and repair/growth of tissues. Proteins (Beef, Chicken, Soy, etc.) are also building blocks of our muscles, bones, cartilage, and skin, otherwise noted as vital! Lean proteins are our best bet! Eggs, Greek yogurt, lentils, and skinned and slim chicken breast are all great choices. Each meal we have should incorporate protein.

Carbs, all those starchy white vegetables, and grains should be kept to a minimum or completely avoided. This includes white bread, white rice, and white potatoes; they have a higher glycemic index (ranking of how they affect blood glucose levels). Processed sugars, of course, are incredibly high on the index. Trans fats, more specifically partially hydrogenated oils, we should avoid altogether. The American Heart Association states that "trans fats raise your bad (LDL) cholesterol levels and lower your good (HDL) cholesterol levels, which increases your risk of developing heart disease and stroke."

There are bad choices, good choices, and great choices of food. We tend to think of vegetables as a great food choice. However, not all vegetables are created equal. This again will be broken down further in part 2. For now, eat your veggies! I feel cruciferous veggies are the healthiest (i.e., cabbage, cauliflower, kale, garden cress, bok choy, broccoli, brussels sprouts, and similar green leafy vegetables). Try to eat a veggie with at least half your meals, preferably all! Healthy fats help lower cholesterol, blood pressure, and the risk of heart disease and strokes. These fats include almonds, avocados, olives, peanut butter, flaxseeds, and more. Also, healthy fats should be incorporated into half of your meals; if you eat veggies in only half of your meals, eat fats in the other half. The discussion of fats leads us to supplementation. There are so many supplements (vitamins, minerals, etc.) to discuss, and we will dive into more details in part 2. The following will discuss a few primary supplements.

Omega-3 fatty acids are polyunsaturated fats and are beneficial to your health. Healthy fats help our health and wellness in many ways. For starters, they help control our blood pressure and cholesterol. Healthy fats can also aid in weight reduction. Healthy fats benefit memory (Omegas), focus and even ease joint pain. Sounds too good to be true? A recent study from 2019 regarding the effects, mechanisms, and clinical relevance of omega-3 fatty acids shows it to have anti-inflammatory actions. As you may recall from reading, inflammation can cause heart disease, diabetes, and more.

We all know that vitamin C is healthy and is a natural antioxidant because it inhibits oxidation (this means it protects cells from potential inflammation). Vitamin C is found naturally in many fruits and vegetables (which fruits and vegetables?) However, do we take in enough? Does it help? Vitamin C's antioxidant function limits damage from free radicals (oxygen and nitrogen) produced during normal cell metabolism and immune activation of neutrophils in response to bacteria, viruses, and toxins (Carr & Maggini, 2017). Vitamin C stimulates neutrophil migration to the infection site in response to chemo-attractants and enhances phagocytosis and oxidant generation, ultimately killing pathogens (Carr & Maggini, 2017). In layman's terms, Vitamin C benefits our immune system. The same study suggests that minimum daily use should be between 100-200mg per day per adult and upwards of a gram daily to combat the body's increased inflammatory response and metabolic demand.

Vitamin D is another essential vitamin! Yes, when we are exposed to the sun, our body creates Vitamin D. How much sun is considered safe? Too much sun leads to skin cancer, yet we need Vitamin D. We need more Vitamin D than our body can produce. The recommended dietary allowance (RDA) for Vitamin D is meager at 400IU to 600IU daily for adults for worries of toxicity, which is far under what is needed. Harvard suggests 2000IU daily is safe, whereas most supplements are 5000IU, which for a healthy individual is also safe!

Why is Vitamin D beneficial? Well, it aids in calcium absorption, thus helping to fight osteoporosis, a condition in which bones become weak. It also helps to regulate cell growth. A recent study by the National Cancer Institute has shown that supplementing with 1000IU per day decreases the risk of cancer death.

Vitamin D is a prohormone created by our kidneys and impacts our immune system. After absorbing Vitamin D, it converts into a calcitriol hormone, which helps absorb calcium. Another significant benefit of Vitamin D is its ability to support and even increase a man's testosterone level. The Division of Endocrinology and Metabolism in Austria reported that 65 men were split into two groups in a year-long study. Half of them took 3,300 IU of vitamin D every day. The supplement group's vitamin D levels doubled, and their testosterone levels increased by around 20%, from 10.7 nmol/l to 13.4 nmol; this is significant! One other thing with vitamin D, it is fat-soluble, meaning it needs to be taken with food (fats).

Coenzyme Q10, aka CoQ10, is another fantastic supplement. CoQ10 has been shown to enhance mitochondria (the powerhouse of our cells) function, which in turn helps to support every cell in the human body. CoQ10 can benefit the brain, heart, and nervous system, asthma, chronic lung disease, diabetes, and the whole metabolic system. CoQ10 has shown great promise in laboratory and animal studies on Alzheimer's disease. By slowing oxidative damage, CoQ10 reduces the deposition of destructive amyloid β-peptide proteins in brain cells (Wadsworth, Bishop, Pappu, Woltjer, & Quinn, 2008). Ubiquinol CoQ10 has been shown to have better bioavailability and should be used at 100mg daily.

With so many supplements on the market, what should you use? Well, quality supplements cost much more than regular supermarket brands. Quality is essential; the facilities used to manufacture the accessories should be GMP certified (good manufacturing practice), which sets recommending manufacturing guidelines. The products from the Life Extension Foundation have a reputation for manufacturing good quality products, and I use them personally. Start supplementing slowly, and remember to listen to your body. Start with a good multi-vitamin, then add as you deem fit!

WELLNESS 101

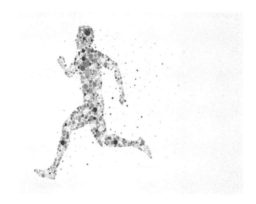

Everyone's body and needs are different; however, these are some basic guidelines:

• **Water = life:** Drink at least a half ounce of water per lb. of your weight! I.e., 120 lbs. = 60 ounces of water, almost 8 cups or four water bottles! Not too hard? (I shoot for a gallon.)

• **Sleep:** Our body recovers and grows when we sleep! In a perfect world, we would get eight quality hours in; however, let's try for at least 6! If we do not sleep enough, our body becomes stressed, which increases inflammation and cortisol levels, which stores fat, especially around the midsection and thighs!

• **Small meals:** Eat every 2.5-4 hours/with quality protein, healthy fats, and low glycemic carbs! A vegetable with each meal is great for many reasons. Shoot for 5-6 small meals a day!

• **Healthy Carbs, veggies, fruits, and whole grains!**

• Keep away from white potatoes, white bread, and white rice. Choose whole wheat, whole grains, sweet potatoes, and, if needed, jasmine or basmati rice!

• **Exercise:** Does not need to be long or vigorous. Every day, we need at least 20 minutes of activity. Swimming, walking, yoga, Pilates, and tennis are excellent choices! Of course, as time passes, you will need to kick it up a notch to help with cardiac output!

This is just a start; remember, it's all about choices!

Supplements:

- Vit D
- Vit C
- Multivitamin
- CoQ10
- Omega 3
- B-Complex

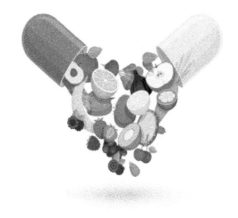

Endnote

To reinvent healthcare and focus on prevention, wellness, and quality of life, we must have a multidisciplinary approach to understanding what causes disease (inflammation), what supports our body (physical and mental support), and our goals.

I hope you enjoyed this beginner's guide (part 1) to functional health and wellness!

Remember to pay attention to your body; it will tell you what is needed. Also, please remember to **Live, Love, Learn, and Teach!**

To stay up to date subscribe at www.Pre-Invent.com.

References:

Boles, A., Kandimalla, R., & Reddy, P. H. (2017). Dynamics of diabetes and obesity: an epidemiological perspective. Biochimica et Biophysica Acta (BBA)-Molecular Basis of Disease, 1863(5), 1026-1036.

Calder, Philip C. "Marine omega-3 fatty acids and inflammatory processes: effects, mechanisms, and clinical relevance." Biochimica et Biophysica Acta (BBA)-Molecular and Cell Biology of Lipids 1851.4 (2015): 469-484.

Cancer Facts and Figures 2023, American Cancer Society.

https://www.cancer.org/content/dam/cancer-org/research/cancer-facts-and-statistics/annual-cancer-facts-and-figures/2023/2023-cancer-facts-and-figures.pdf.

Carr, A. C., & Maggini, S. (2017). Vitamin C and immune function. Nutrients, 9(11), 1211.

Durrani, H. (2016). Healthcare and healthcare systems: inspiring progress and prospects. Health, 2.

Farjadian, S., Moghtaderi, M., Kalani, M., Gholami, T., & Teshnizi, S. H. (2016). Effects of omega-3 fatty acids on serum levels of T-helper cytokines in children with asthma. *Cytokine, 85*, 61-66.

Genes play a key role in Exercise Outcomes -- ScienceDaily. (2021, October 14). https://www.sciencedaily.com/releases/2021/10/211014142032.htm

Jones, D. S. (2010). Textbook of functional medicine. Institute for Functional Medicine.

Lagua, R. T., & Claudio, V. S. (2012). Nutrition and diet therapy reference dictionary. Springer Science & Business Media.

Li, K., Huang, T., Zheng, J., Wu, K., & Li, D. (2014). Effect of marine-derived n-3 polyunsaturated fatty acids on C-reactive protein, interleukin six and tumor necrosis factor α: a meta-analysis. *PloS one, 9*(2), e88103.

Pilz, S., Frisch, S., Koertke, H., Kuhn, J., Dreier, J., Obermayer-Pietsch, B., ... & Zittermann, A. (2011). Effect of vitamin D supplementation on testosterone levels in men. Hormone and Metabolic Research, 43(03), 223-225.

Sawi i, T., Ruszkowska, M., Danielewicz, A., Niedźwiedzka, E., Arłukowicz, T., & Przybyłowicz, K. E. (2021). A review of colorectal cancer in terms of epidemiology, risk factors, development, symptoms and diagnosis. *Cancers, 13*(9), 2025.

Wadsworth, T. L., Bishop, J. A., Pappu, A. S., Woltjer, R. L., & Quinn, J. F. (2008). Evaluation of coenzyme Q as an antioxidant strategy for Alzheimer's disease. Journal of Alzheimer's Disease, 14(2), 225-234.

https://www.cdc.gov/nchs/fastats/health-expenditures.htm

https://www.who.int/about/who-we-are/frequently-asked-questions

https://www.eupati.eu/glossary/physical-health/

https://www.medicalnewstoday.com/articles/150999.php

https://shcs.ucdavis.edu/wellness/what-is-wellness

https://www.ifm.org/functional-medicine/what-is-functional-medicine/

https://wa.kaiserpermanente.org/kbase/topic.jhtml?docId=ad1169

https://my.clevelandclinic.org/health/articles/9476-fad-diets

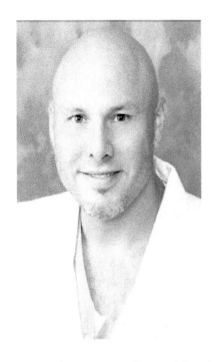

Steve is an experienced healthcare professional with a background in sports nutrition, nursing, and education. Steve has dedicated close to twenty years to researching and developing a comprehensive approach to healthcare that prioritizes prevention and overall wellbeing. Even at an early age as a youth athlete and later in college, coaching youth sports; health and wellness has been a passion for him!

With a "Master of Science in Nursing" as well as achieving "Certified Nurse-Operating Room (CNOR)," his years of extensive research and experiences have shaped his perspective on healthcare, emphasizing the importance of mental, physical, spiritual, emotional, and financial well-being in achieving overall health. Through these years of research and experience, Steve understands the significance of lifestyle choices, nutrition, supplementation, and personalized approaches to wellness.

Steve is a passionate person and is committed to helping individuals reinvent their approach to health and wellness by promoting a multidisciplinary and holistic view of healthcare.

Steve's dedication to educating and empowering individuals to take charge of their health shines through in his everyday dealings, making him a valuable contributor to the field of health and wellness. #LiveLoveLearnandTeach

Printed in the USA
CPSIA information can be obtained
at www.ICGtesting.com
LVHW021446210124
769172LV00060B/1042

9 798218 341039